Instant Pot Breakfast Cookbook for Families

Best Breakfast Recipes Made Simple

Samantha Walker

Sommario

Sommario

Introduction

This complete and useful guide to instant pot cooking with over 1000 recipes for breakfast, dinner, supper, and even desserts! This is one of the most comprehensive instant pot cookbooks ever published thanks to its variety and accurate instructions.

Innovative recipes and classics, modern take on family's most loved meals – all this is tasty, simple and of course as healthy as it can be. Change the way you cook with these innovative instant pot instructions. Need a new dinner or a dessert? Here you are! Best instant pot meals come together in a few simple steps, even a beginner can do it! The instant pot defines the way you cook every day. This instant pot cookbook helps you make the absolute most out of your weekly menu.

The only instant pot book you will ever need with the ultimate collection of recipes will aid you towards a simpler and healthier kitchen experience. If you want to save time cooking meals more efficiently, if you want to offer your family food that can satisfy even the pickiest eater, you are in the right place! Master your instant pot and make your cooking needs fit into your busy lifestyle

Breakfast recipes

Fragrant Coffee

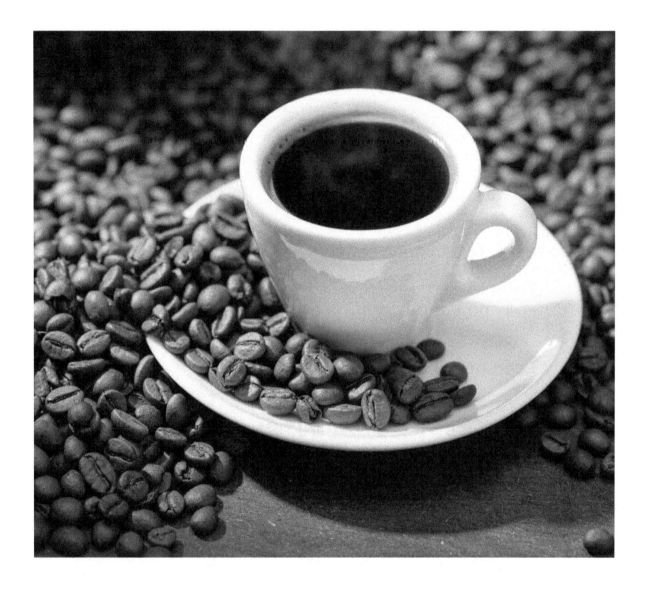

Prep time: 10 minutes

Cooking time: 5 minutes

Servings: 4

Ingredients:

- 4 teaspoon butter

- 2 cups of water

- 4 teaspoons instant coffee

- 1 tablespoon Erythritol

- 1/3 cup heavy cream

- 1 teaspoon ground cinnamon

- ½ teaspoon vanilla extract

Directions:

1. Pour water, heavy cream, ground cinnamon, and vanilla extract in the cooker.

2. Add instant coffee and stir well until homogenous.

3. Close and seal the lid.

4. Cook the coffee mixture on high-pressure mode for 4 minutes.

5. Then allow natural pressure release for 10 minutes.

6. Open the lid and add butter. Stir well and pour coffee in the serving cups.

Nutrition: calories 71, fat 7.5, fiber 0.3, carbs 0.8, protein 0.3

Veggie Egg Cups

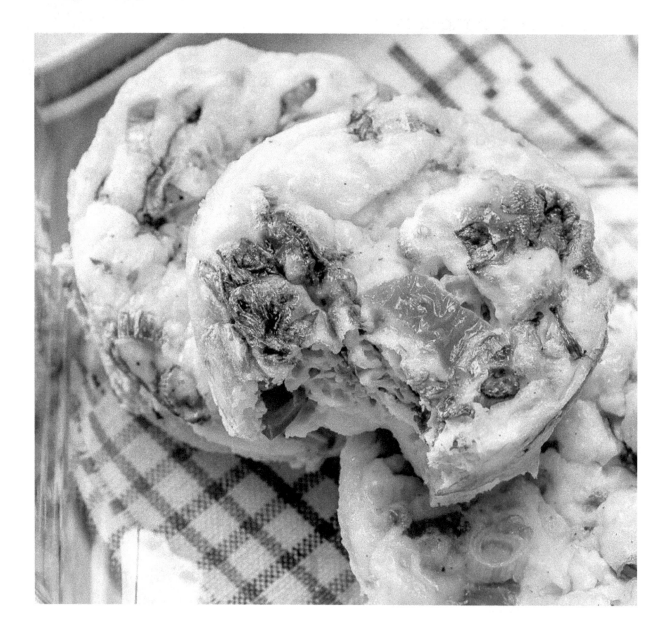

Prep time: 5 minutes

Cooking time: 7 minutes

Servings: 4

Ingredients:

- 1 zucchini

- 2 tablespoon almond flour

- ½ teaspoon salt

- 1 teaspoon butter

- 4 eggs

Directions:

1. Grate zucchini and mix it up with almond flour and salt.

2. Spread the muffin molds with butter and place grated zucchini inside in the shape of nests.

3. Then beat eggs inside "zucchini nests" and place them in the cooker.

4. Lower the air fryer lid.

5. Cook the zucchini cups for 7 minutes.

6. When the eggs are solid, the meal is cooked.

Nutrition: calories 99, fat 7.2, fiber 0.9, carbs 2.7, protein 6.9

Egg Fluffs

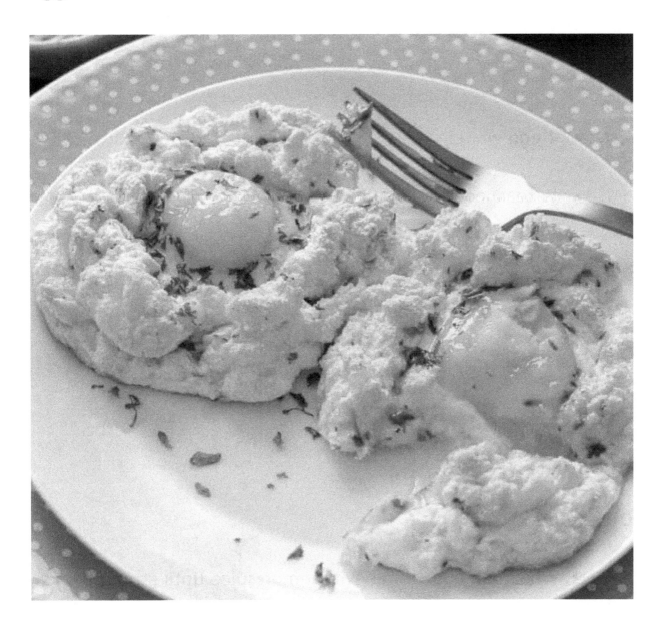

Prep time: 10 minutes

Cooking time: 6 minutes

Servings: 4

Ingredients:

- 4 egg whites

- ½ teaspoon lemon juice

- ½ teaspoon salt

- 1 teaspoon almond flour

Directions:

1. Whisk the egg whites with lemon juice until strong peaks.

2. Add salt and almond flour. Stir it.

3. Place the egg white clouds in the cooker with the help of the spoon.

4. Lower the air fryer lid.

5. Cook the egg clouds for 6 minutes or until they are light brown.

Nutrition: calories 21, fat 0.4, fiber 0.1, carbs 0.4, protein 3.7

Avocado Bacon Bombs

Prep time: 10 minutes

Cooking time: 10 minutes

Servings: 4

Ingredients:

- 1 avocado, peeled, cored

- 4 oz bacon, sliced

- 1 tablespoon almond flour

- 1 tablespoon flax meal

- ½ teaspoon salt

Directions:

1. Blend together avocado, almond flour, flax meal, and salt.

2. When the mixture is smooth, transfer it in the mixing bowl.

3. Make the medium size balls from it and wrap in the bacon.

4. Secure the balls with the toothpicks.

5. After this, transfer the bombs in the cooker and ser air crisp mode.

6. Close the lid and cook the meal for 10 minutes.

Nutrition: calories 303, fat 25.8, fiber 4.6, carbs 6.7, protein 13.3

Pepper Avocado

Prep time: 15 minutes

Cooking time: 10 minutes

Servings: 2

Ingredients:

- 1 avocado, halved

- 2 eggs

- ½ teaspoon ground black pepper

- 1 teaspoon butter

Directions:

1. Beat the eggs in the avocado halves, sprinkle with ground black pepper.

2. Then add butter.

3. Add 1 cup of water in the cooker.

4. Transfer the avocado halves on the trivet in the Foodi Pressure cooker and close the lid.

5. Cook the breakfast for 10 minutes on High-pressure mode.

6. Then allow natural pressure release for 10 minutes.

Nutrition: calories 286, fat 25.2, fiber 6.9, carbs 9.3, protein 7.5

Creamy Omelet

Prep time: 10 minutes

Cooking time: 7 minutes

Servings: 4

Ingredients:

- 4 eggs, whisked

- ¼ cup cream

- ½ teaspoon salt

- 2 oz bacon, chopped

- 1 teaspoon butter, melted

- 1 cup water, for cooking

Directions:

1. Mix up together whisked eggs, cream, salt, and chopped bacon.

2. Add melted butter and stir the mixture.

3. Pour egg mixture in the mason jars.

4. Pour 1 cup of water in the Pressure cooker and insert trivet.

5. Place mason jars on the trivet.

6. Close the lid and cook an omelet for 7 minutes on High-pressure mode.

7. Then use quick pressure release. Chill the meal little before serving.

Nutrition: calories 234, fat 18, fiber 0, carbs 1.2, protein 16.2

Flax Pancake

Prep time: 10 minutes

Cooking time: 10 minutes

Servings: 2

Ingredients:

- 7 oz cauliflower

- 2 eggs, whisked

- 2 tablespoons almond flour

- 1 tablespoon flax meal

- 1 teaspoon butter

- 1 teaspoon chili flakes

- 1 teaspoon dried dill

Directions:

1. Grind the cauliflower and mix it up with the whisked eggs, almond flour, flax meal, chili flakes, and dried dill.

2. Stir the mixture well.

3. Preheat Foodi cooker on saute mode and add butter. Melt it.

4. Place cauliflower mixture in the cooker with the help of the spoon (to get pancake shape) and cook for 4 minutes from each side.

Nutrition: calories 161, fat 11.2, fiber 4.3, carbs 8.4, protein 9.9

Almond Eggs

Prep time: 5 minutes

Cooking time: 9 minutes

Servings: 5

Ingredients:

- 7 eggs

- ½ cup almond milk

- 1 tablespoon butter

- 1 teaspoon basil

- ¼ cup fresh parsley

- 1 teaspoon salt

- 1 teaspoon paprika

- 4 ounces sliced bacon

- 1 tablespoon cilantro

Directions:

1. Beat the eggs in a mixing bowl and whisk well.

2. Add the almond milk, basil, salt, paprika, and cilantro. Stir the mixture well.

3. Chop the bacon and parsley.

4. Set the pressure cooker mode to "Sauté" and add the bacon. Cook it for 3 minutes.

5. Add the whisked egg mixture, and cook for 5 additional minutes.

6. Stir the eggs carefully using a wooden spoon or spatula.

7. Sprinkle the eggs with the chopped parsley, and cook it for 4 minutes.

8. When the eggs are cooked, remove them from the pressure cooker.

Nutrition: calories 289, fat 23.7, fiber 0.8, carbs 2.6, protein 16.9

Avocado Eggs

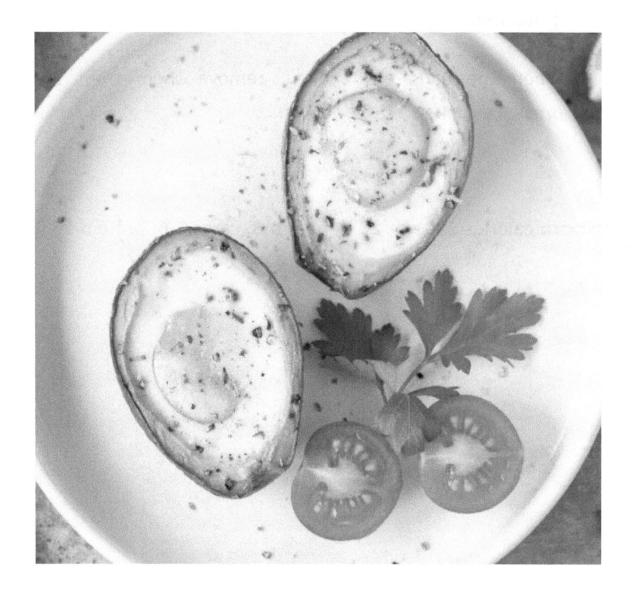

Prep time: 15 minutes

Cooking time: 15 minutes

Servings: 6

Ingredients:

- 2 cups of water

- 1 avocado, pittcd

- 4 eggs

- 1 teaspoon paprika

- ½ teaspoon ground black pepper

- 1 sweet bell pepper

- 1 teaspoon salt

- 3 tablespoons heavy cream

- 3 ounces lettuce leaves

Directions:

1. Put the eggs and water in the pressure cooker and close the lid.

2. Set the pressure cooker mode to "Pressure," and cook for 15 minutes.

3. Remove the eggs from the pressure cooker, and transfer them to an ice bath.

4. Chop the avocado, and remove the seeds from bell pepper.

5. Dice the bell peppers and Peel the eggs and chop them.

6. Combine the chopped ingredients together in a mixing bowl.

7. Sprinkle the mixture with the paprika, ground black pepper, salt, and stir.

8. Transfer the mixture in the lettuce leaves, sprinkle them with the cream, and serve.

Nutrition: calories 168, fat 12.9, fiber 3, carbs 6.75, protein 7

Cheddar Migas

Prep time: 10 minutes

Cooking time: 10 minutes

Servings: 6

Ingredients:

- 10 eggs

- 1 jalapeno pepper

- 8 ounces tomatoes

- 1 tablespoon chicken stock

- 7 ounces cheddar cheese

- 2 white onions

- 2 cups tortilla chips

- 1 sweet bell pepper

- ½ cup beef stock

- 1 teaspoon salt

Directions:

1. Whisk the eggs in the mixing bowl.

2. Chop the jalapeno peppers and tomatoes.

3. Grate the cheddar cheese.

4. Peel the onions and chop them.

5. Crush the tortilla chips. Chop the bell peppers.

6. Combine the jalapeno pepper, tomatoes, onion, and chopped bell pepper together and stir the mixture.

7. Set the pressure cooker mode to "Sauté", and transfer the vegetable mixture.

8. Cook it for 5 minutes.

9. Add the whisked eggs mixture.

10.   Add the stocks, salt, and grated cheese. Mix up the mixture well, and cook it for 4 minutes.

11.   Add the crushed tortilla chips, and cook for 1 minute more.

12.   Stir it and serve.

13.   Note: Only add salt if using low-sodium chicken and beef stock; otherwise, you can omit the salt.!

Nutrition: calories 295, fat 19.3, fiber 1, carbs 9.27, protein 21

Soft Eggs

Prep time: 7 minutes

Cooking time: 7 minutes

Servings: 4

Ingredients:

- 7 ounces sliced bacon

- 4 eggs, boiled

- 1 teaspoon cilantro

- ½ cup spinach

- 2 teaspoons butter

- ½ teaspoon ground white pepper

- 3 tablespoons heavy cream

Directions:

1. Lay the bacon flat and sprinkle it with the ground white pepper and cilantro on both sides of the slices and stir the mixture.

2. Peel the eggs, and wrap them in the spinach leaves.

3. Wrap the eggs in the sliced bacon.

4. Set the pressure cooker mode to "Sauté" and transfer the wrapped eggs.

5. Add butter and cook for 10 minutes.

6. When the cooking time ends, remove the eggs from the pressure cooker and sprinkle them with the cream.

7. Serve the dish immediately.

Nutrition: calories 325, fat 28.4, fiber 2, carbs 5.24, protein 15

Creamy Soufflé

Prep time: 10 minutes

Cooking time: 20 minutes

Servings: 6

Ingredients:

- 3 eggs

- 1 cup cream

- 6 ounces of cottage cheese

- 4 tablespoons butter

- ⅓ cup dried apricots

- 1 tablespoon sour cream

- 2 tablespoons sugar

- 1 teaspoon vanilla extract

Directions:

1. Whisk the eggs and combine them with cream.

2. Transfer the cottage cheese to a mixing bowl, and mix it well using a hand mixer.

3. Add the whisked eggs, butter, sour cream, sugar, and vanilla extract.

4. Blend the mixture well until smooth.

5. Add the apricots, and stir the mixture well.

6. Transfer the soufflé in the pressure cooker and close the lid. Set the pressure cooker mode to «Sauté», and cook for 20 minutes.

7. When the cooking time ends, let the soufflé cool little and serve.

Nutrition: calories 266, fat 21.1, fiber 1, carbs 11.72, protein 8

Zucchini Casserole

Prep time: 10 minutes

Cooking time: 30 minutes

Servings: 8

Ingredients:

- 6 ounces cheddar cheese

- 1 zucchini

- ½ cup ground chicken

- 4 ounces Parmesan cheese

- 3 tablespoons butter

- 1 teaspoon paprika

- 1 teaspoon salt

- 1 teaspoon basil

- 1 teaspoon cilantro

- ½ cup fresh dill

- ⅓ cup tomato juice

- ½ cup cream

- 2 red sweet bell peppers

Directions:

1. Grate cheddar cheese.

2. Chop the zucchini and combine it with the ground chicken.

3. Sprinkle the mixture with the paprika, salt, basil, cilantro, tomato juice, and cream. Stir the mixture well. Transfer it to the pressure cooker.

4. Chop the dill, sprinkle the mixture in the pressure cooker, and add the butter. Chop the Parmesan cheese and add it to the pressure cooker.

5. Chop the bell peppers and add them too. Sprinkle the mixture with the grated cheddar cheese and close the lid.

6. Set the pressure cooker mode to "Sauté", and cook for 30 minutes.

7. When the cooking time ends, let the casserole chill briefly and serve.

Nutrition: calories 199, fat 14.7, fiber 1, carbs 6.55, protein 11

Spinach Casserole

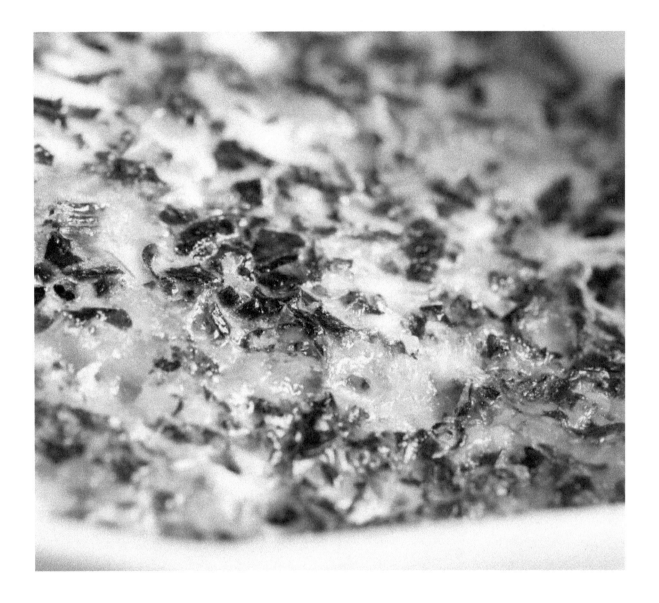

Prep time: 6 minutes

Cooking time: 6 minutes

Servings: 5

Ingredients:

- 2 cups spinach

- 8 eggs

- ½ cup almond milk

- 1 teaspoon salt

- 1 tablespoon olive oil

- 1 teaspoon ground black pepper

- 4 ounces Parmesan cheese

Directions:

1. Add the eggs to a mixing bowl and whisk them.

2. Chop the spinach and add it to the egg mixture.

3. Add the almond milk, salt, olive oil, and ground black pepper. Stir the mixture well. Transfer the egg mixture to the pressure cooker and close the lid.

4. Set the pressure cooker mode to "Steam," and cook for 6 minutes.

5. Grate the cheese. When the cooking time ends, remove the omelet from the pressure cooker and transfer it to a serving plate.

6. Sprinkle the dish with the grated cheese and serve.

Nutrition: calories 257, fat 20.4, fiber 0.9, carbs 3.4, protein 17.1

Spicy Romano Bites

Prep time: 6 minutes

Cooking time: 20 minutes

Servings: 8

Ingredients:

- 10 ounces Romano cheese

- 6 ounces sliced bacon

- 1 teaspoon oregano

- 5 ounces puff pastry

- 1 teaspoon butter

- 2 egg yolks

- 1 teaspoon sesame seeds

Directions:

1. Chop Romano cheese into small cubes.

2. Roll the puff pastry using a rolling pin. Whisk the egg yolks.

3. Sprinkle them with the oregano and sesame seeds.

4. Cut the puff pastry into the squares, and place an equal amount of butter on every square. Wrap the cheese cubes in the sliced bacon.

5. Place the wrapped cheese cubes onto the puff pastry squares. Make the "bites" of the dough and brush them with the egg yolk mixture.

6. Transfer the bites in the pressure cooker.

7. Close the lid, and set the pressure cooker mode to "Steam." Cook for 20 minutes.

8. When the cooking time ends, remove the dish from the pressure cooker and place on a serving dish.

Nutrition: calories 321, fat 24.4, fiber 1, carbs 10.9, protein 16

Eggs and Chives

Prep time: 4 minutes

Cooking time: 4 minutes

Servings: 3

Ingredients:

- 3 eggs

- 6 ounces ham

- 1 teaspoon salt

- ½ teaspoon ground white pepper

- 1 teaspoon paprika

- ¼ teaspoon ground ginger

- 2 tablespoons chives

Directions:

1. Take three small ramekins and coat them with vegetable oil spray.

2. Beat the eggs add an equal amount to the ramekins. Sprinkle the eggs with the salt, ground black pepper, and paprika.

3. Transfer the ramekins to the pressure cooker and set the mode to "Steam."

4. Close the lid, and cook for 4 minutes. Meanwhile, chop the ham and chives and combine them.

5. Add ground ginger and stir into the ham mixture well. Transfer the mixture to the serving plates.

6. When the cooking time ends, remove the eggs from the pressure cooker and put them atop the ham mixture.

Nutrition: calories 205, fat 11.1, fiber 1, carbs 6.47, protein 19

Zucchini Quiche

Prep time: 15 minutes

Cooking time: 40 minutes

Servings: 6

Ingredients:

- 3 green zucchini

- 7 ounces puff pastry

- 2 onions

- 1 cup dill

- 2 eggs

- 3 tablespoons butter

- ½ cup cream

- 6 ounces cheddar cheese

- 1 teaspoon salt

- 1 teaspoon paprika

Directions:

1. Wash the zucchini and grate the vegetables.

2. Peel the onions and chop them. Grate the cheddar cheese.

3. Whisk the eggs in the mixing bowl. Roll out the puff pastry.

4. Spread the pressure cooker basket with the butter and transfer the dough to there.

5. Add grated zucchini and chopped onions, and sprinkle the vegetable mixture with the salt and paprika.

6. Chop the dill and add it to the quiche. Sprinkle the dish with the grated cheese and egg mixture, and pour the cream on top.

7. Close the pressure cooker lid, and set the mode to "Steam."

8. Cook the quiche for 40 minutes.

9. When the cooking time ends, check if the dish is cooked and remove it from the pressure cooker. Let the dish cool briefly and serve.

Nutrition: calories 398, fat 28.4, fiber 2, carbs 25.82, protein 12

Almond Pumpkin Cook

Prep time: 10 minutes

Cooking time: 15 minutes

Servings: 5

Ingredients:

- 1 cup almond milk

- 1 cup of water

- 1 pound pumpkin

- 1 teaspoon cinnamon

- ½ teaspoon cardamom

- ½ teaspoon turmeric

- ⅓ cup coconut flakes

- 2 teaspoons Erythritol

Directions:

1. Peel the pumpkin and chop it roughly.

2. Transfer the chopped pumpkin in the pressure cooker and add almond milk and water. Sprinkle the mixture with the cinnamon, cardamom, turmeric, and Erythritol.

3. Add coconut flakes and stir the mixture well.

4. Close the pressure cooker lid, and set the mode to "Sauté." Cook for 15 minutes.

5. When the cooking time ends, blend the mixture until smooth using a hand blender.

6. Ladle the pumpkin in the serving bowls and serve.

Nutrition: calories 163, fat 13.5, fiber 4.5, carbs 13.1, protein 2.3

Tomato Omelet

Prep time: 8 minutes

Cooking time: 9 minutes

Servings: 6

Ingredients:

- 5 eggs

- ½ cup of coconut milk

- 4 tablespoons tomato paste

- 1 teaspoon salt

- 1 tablespoon turmeric

- ½ cup cilantro

- 1 tablespoon butter

- 4 ounces Parmesan cheese

Directions:

1. Whisk the eggs with the coconut milk and tomato paste in the mixing bowl.

2. Add salt and turmeric and stir the mixture. Grate the Parmesan cheese and add it to the egg mixture.

3. Mince the cilantro and add it to the egg mixture. Add the butter in the pressure cooker and pour in the egg mixture.

4. Close the pressure cooker lid, and set the mode to "Steam."

5. Cook for 9 minutes. Open the pressure cooker to let the omelet rest. Transfer it to serving plates and enjoy.

Nutrition: calories 189, fat 14.6, fiber 1.2, carbs 4.9, protein 11.7

Poached Eggs with Paprika

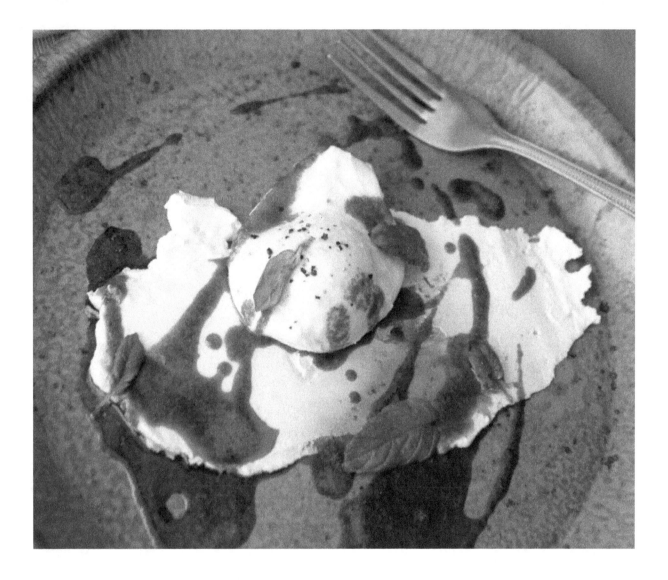

Prep time: 5 minutes

Cooking time: 5 minutes

Servings: 4

Ingredients:

- 4 eggs

- 3 medium tomatoes

- 1 red onion

- 1 teaspoon salt

- 1 tablespoon olive oil

- ½ teaspoon white pepper

- ½ teaspoon paprika

- 1 tablespoon fresh dill

Directions:

1. Spray the ramekins with the olive oil inside. Beat the eggs in a mixing bowl and add an equal amount to each ramekin.

2. Combine the paprika, white pepper, fresh dill, and salt together in a mixing bowl and stir the mixture.

3. Dice the red onion and tomatoes and combine. Add the seasonings and stir the mixture.

4. Sprinkle the eggs with the tomato mixture. Transfer the eggs to the pressure cooker.

5. Close the lid, and set the pressure cooker mode to "Steam". Cook for 5 minutes.

6. Remove the dish from the pressure cooker and rest briefly. Let it rest for a few minutes and dish immediately.

Nutrition: calories 194, fat 13.5, fiber 2, carbs 8.45, protein 10

Poultry Burrito

Prep time: 10 minutes

Cooking time: 45 minutes

Servings: 6

Ingredients:

- 6 large almond flour tortillas (keto tortillas)

- 1 pound chicken

- ½ cup chicken stock

- 1 tablespoon tomato paste

- 1 teaspoon sour cream

- 1 teaspoon ground black pepper

- ½ teaspoon paprika

- 1 teaspoon cilantro

- ½ teaspoon turmeric

- 1 white onion

- 2 sweet bell peppers

- ½ cup cauliflower rice

- 1 cup of water

Directions:

1. Chop the chicken roughly and transfer it to the pressure cooker. Add chicken stock, tomato paste, sour cream, and water.

2. Sprinkle the mixture with the ground black pepper, paprika, cilantro, and turmeric. Peel the onion, and remove the seeds from the bell peppers.

3. Dice onion and peppers and set aside. Sprinkle the pressure cooker mixture with the cauliflower rice and close the lid.

4. Set the pressure cooker mode to "Steam," and cook for 30 minutes.

5. Add the chopped onion and peppers and cook for 15 minutes.

6. When the cooking time ends, shred the chicken and transfer the mixture to the tortillas.

7. Wrap the tortillas and serve the dish immediately.

Nutrition: calories 295, fat 10.8, fiber 5.2, carbs 14.3, protein 35.1

Stuffed Buns with Egg

Prep time: 8 minutes

Cooking time: 10 minutes

Servings: 6

Ingredients:

- 3 large keto bread rolls

- 4 eggs

- 7 ounces cheddar cheese

- 1 teaspoon salt

- ½ teaspoon red chili flakes

- ½ teaspoon sour cream

- 1 tablespoon butter

Directions:

1. Cut the keto bread rolls in half. Hollow out the center of the bread half partially.

2. Combine the salt, pepper flakes, and sour cream together and stir gently. Add the eggs to a mixing bowl and whisk.

3. Add the butter in the pressure cooker. Pour the eggs equally into the keto bread roll halves.

4. Transfer the bread in the pressure cooker. Sprinkle the dish with the spice mixture.

5. Grate the cheddar cheese and sprinkle the bread with the grated cheese. Close the lid, and set the pressure cooker mode to "Steam." Cook for 10 minutes.

6. Let the dish rest before serving it.

Nutrition: calories 259, fat 19.2, fiber 3.6, carbs 2.6, protein 17.5

Coconut Frittata

Prep time: 10 minutes

Cooking time: 10 minutes

Servings: 6

Ingredients:

- 7 eggs

- ½ cup of coconut milk

- 1 teaspoon salt

- ½ teaspoon paprika

- ½ cup parsley

- 8 ounces ham

- 1 teaspoon white pepper

- 1 tablespoon lemon zest

- 1 teaspoon olive oil

- 1 tomato

Directions:

1. Beat the eggs in the mixing bowl.

2. Add coconut milk, salt, paprika, white pepper, and lemon zest. Blend the mixture well using a hand mixer.

3. Chop the tomato and add it to the egg mixture.

4. Chop the ham, and top the egg mixture with the ham. Stir it carefully until smooth. Chop the parsley.

5. Spray the pressure cooker with the olive oil inside.

6. Transfer the egg mixture in the pressure cooker.

7. Sprinkle it with the chopped parsley and close the lid.

8. Cook the frittata for 10 minutes at the mode to "Steam."

9. When the time is cooked, let cooked, let the dish cool little and serve.

Nutrition: calories 193, fat 14, fiber 1.4, carbs 4.2, protein 13.5

Zucchini Frittata

Prep time: 10 minutes

Cooking time: 15 minutes

Servings: 6

Ingredients:

- 10 eggs

- 1 cup of coconut milk

- 1 teaspoon salt

- ½ teaspoon ground black pepper

- 1 sweet bell pepper

- ½ jalapeno pepper

- 3 tomatoes

- 1 zucchini

- 1 tablespoon butter

- 5 ounces asparagus

- ½ cup cilantro

Directions:

1. Beat the eggs in the mixing bowl until combined.

2. Add the coconut milk and butter and combine. Sprinkle the mixture with the salt and, ground black pepper and mix well.

3. Chop the zucchini, tomatoes, asparagus, and cilantro.

4. Remove the seeds from the bell pepper and chop it. Slice the jalapeno pepper.

5. Transfer the egg mixture to the pressure cooker.

6. Top with the vegetables and cilantro.

7. Close the lid, and set the pressure cooker mode to "Steam." Cook for 15 minutes.

8. Remove the frittata from the pressure cooker. Serve immediately.

Nutrition: calories 145, fat 11.4, fiber 1.7, carbs 5.4, protein 7.1

Feta Peppers

Prep time: 10 minutes

Cooking time: 15 minutes

Servings: 3

Ingredients:

- 4 eggs, boiled

- 9 ounces feta cheese

- 1 tablespoon butter

- 2 sweet bell peppers

- 1 teaspoon salt

- 1 cup chicken stock

- ½ cup cilantro

- 1 teaspoon heavy cream

- 2 tablespoons sour cream

- 1 tablespoon tomato paste

Directions:

1. Remove the seeds from the bell peppers.

2. Peel the eggs, and stuff the bell peppers with the eggs. Chop the feta cheese and cilantro and combine them together.

3. Sprinkle the cheese mixture with the salt, cream, sour cream, and tomato paste. Blend the mixture together until smooth.

4. Add the cream mixture to the bell peppers.

5. Add the butter in the pressure cooker, and transfer the stuffed peppers to the pot. Add chicken stock and close the lid.

6. Set the pressure cooker mode to "Steam," and cook for 15 minutes. When the cooking time ends, let the dish rest briefly.

Nutrition: calories 513, fat 37.2, fiber 1, carbs 17.23, protein 28

Soy Eggs

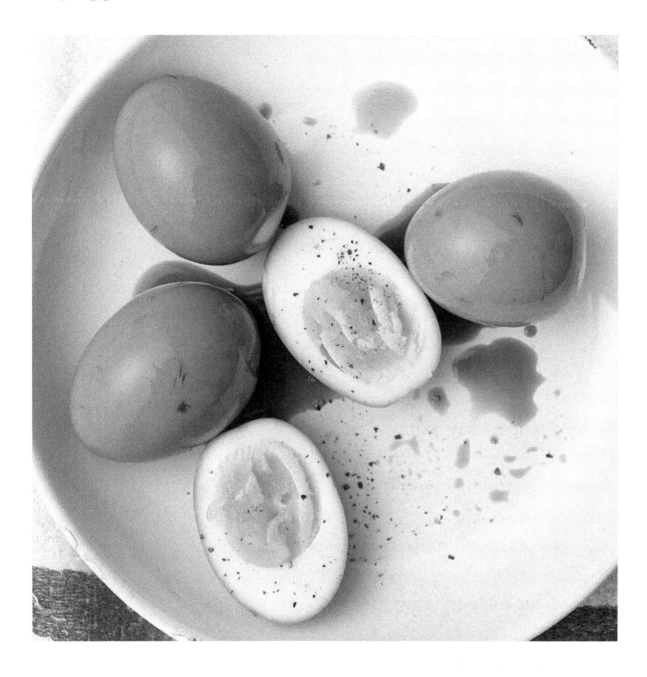

Prep time: 10 minutes

Cooking time: 5 minutes

Servings: 5

Ingredients:

- 1 teaspoon red chili flakes

- ½ cup of water

- 5 eggs, boiled

- 1 teaspoon salt

- ⅓ cup of soy sauce

- 1 teaspoon cilantro

- ½ teaspoon ground black pepper

- 1 tablespoon lemon juice

- 1 tablespoon sugar

- 2 tablespoons mirin

Directions:

1. Peel the eggs, and transfer them to the pressure cooker.

2. Combine the water, chili flakes, salt, soy sauce, cilantro, ground black pepper, lemon juice, and mirin in a mixing bowl.

3. Stir the mixture well until smooth, then pour the mixture in the pressure cooker. Stir it gently, close the lid, and set the pressure cooker mode to "Sauté".

4. Cook for 5 minutes. Transfer the mixture to casserole dish and let it cool.

5. When the eggs are cool, serve them right away and store in the refrigerator to serve later.

Nutrition: calories 189, fat 12.8, fiber 1, carbs 7.7, protein 10

Sweet Cauliflower Rice

Prep time: 10 minutes

Cooking time: 30 minutes

Servings: 3

Ingredients:

- 1 cup cauliflower rice

- 1 cup heavy cream

- 1 cup of coconut milk

- ¼ cup of water

- 1 teaspoon salt

- 4 tablespoons Erythritol

- 1 teaspoon cinnamon

Directions:

1. Pour cream, coconut milk, and water in the pressure cooker.

2. Stir the mixture gently and add salt, Erythritol, and cinnamon.

3. Blend the mixture gently until you mixed well. Add cauliflower rice.

4. Close the pressure cooker lid, and set the mode to "." Cook for 30 minutes.

5. When the cooking time ends, open the lid and stir the mixture gently. Transfer the cooked dish to serving bowls and serve hot.

Nutrition: calories 343, fat 34.5, fiber 2.2, carbs 8.4, protein 4

Morning Cauliflower Rice

Prep time: 10 minutes

Cooking time: 40 minutes

Servings: 7

Ingredients:

- 7 ounces sliced bacon

- 2 cups cauliflower rice

- 1 tablespoon olive oil

- 1 onion

- 4 cups chicken stock

- 1 teaspoon butter

- 1 teaspoon basil

- 1 teaspoon oregano

- 1 teaspoon thyme

Directions:

1. Chop the bacon and transfer it to the pressure cooker. Close the lid, and set the pressure cooker mode to "Sauté", and cook the bacon for 4 minutes.

2. Open the lid and add the cauliflower rice. Sprinkle the mixture with the olive oil and stir. Add chicken stock, butter, basil, oregano, and thyme.

3. Peel the onion and chop it. Sprinkle the cauliflower rice with the chopped onion, mix well, and close the lid.

4. Set the pressure cooker mode to "," and cook for 40 minutes.

5. When the dish is cooked, remove the cauliflower rice from the pressure cooker and stir. Transfer the dish to serving plates and serve.

Nutrition: calories 273, fat 19.6, fiber 8, carbs 25.03, protein 11

Chia Slow Cook

Prep time: 5 minutes

Cooking time: 5 minutes

Servings: 4

Ingredients:

- 1 cup Greek yogurt

- 1 cup of water

- 1 cup chia seeds

- 1 tablespoon liquid stevia

- ½ teaspoon cinnamon

- 1 teaspoon lemon zest

- 2 apples

- ¼ teaspoon salt

- 1 teaspoon clove

Directions:

1. Combine the water and Greek yogurt together and blend well.

2. Transfer the liquid mixture in the pressure cooker and add chia seeds.

3. Stir the mixture and sprinkle it with the liquid stevia, cinnamon, lemon zest, salt, and cloves.

4. Peel the apples and chop them into small chunks.

5. Add the chopped apple in the pressure cooker and stir well. Close the lid, and set the pressure cooker mode to "Steam."

6. Cook for 7 minutes.

7. When the dish is cooked, remove it from the pressure cooker and mix well gently. Serve the chia hot. Enjoy.

Nutrition: calories 259, fat 13.3, fiber 12.8, carbs 29.5, protein 8.5

Ham Cups

Prep time: 5 minutes

Cooking time: 3 minutes

Servings: 4

Ingredients:

- 4 big tomatoes

- 4 eggs

- 7 ounces ham

- 1 tablespoon chives

- 1 teaspoon mayonnaise

- ½ teaspoon butter

- 4 ounces Parmesan cheese

- ½ teaspoon salt

Directions:

1. Wash the tomatoes and remove the flesh, jelly, and seeds from them and add to a mixing bowl.

2. Chop the ham and chives.

3. Combine the chopped ham, chives, and tomato pieces together in a mixing bowl.

4. Add mayonnaise, butter, and salt to the ham mixture and blend well. Grate the Parmesan cheese and beat the eggs in the empty tomato cups.

5. Fill the cups with the ham mixture.

6. Sprinkle them with the grated cheese.

7. Wrap the tomato cups in aluminum foil and transfer them in the pressure cooker.

8. Close the lid, and set the pressure cooker mode to "Sauté." Cook for 10 minutes.

9. When the cooking time ends, remove the tomatoes from the pressure cooker and allow them to rest. Discard the foil and serve immediately.

Nutrition: calories 335, fat 19.8, fiber 1, carbs 12.17, protein 27

Breakfast Creamy Casserole

Prep time: 15 minutes

Cooking time: 30 minutes

Servings: 6

Ingredients:

- 1 pound chicken breast fillets

- 4 egg yolks

- 1 onion

- 1 cup cream

- 10 ounces cheddar cheese

- 1 tablespoon butter

Breakfast Creamy Cacao

Prep time: 5 minutes

Cooking time: 15 minutes

Servings: 2

Ingredients:

- 1 cup heavy cream

- ½ cup of water

- 1 tablespoon cocoa powder

- 1 teaspoon butter

- 1 tablespoon Erythritol

Directions:

1. In the mixing bowl mix up together cocoa powder and heavy cream. When the liquid is smooth, pour it in the instant pot bowl.

2. Add water and sauté the liquid for 5 minutes.

3. After this, add butter and Erythritol. Stir well.

4. Saute the hot cacao for 10 minutes more.

Nutrition value/serving: calories 153, fat 16.3, fiber 0.5, carbs 7.1, protein 1.2

Zucchini Turmeric Fritters

Prep time: 10 minutes

Cooking time: 10 minutes

Servings: 4

Ingredients:

- 2 zucchini, grated

- 1/3 cup Mozzarella, shredded

- 1 egg, beaten

- 2 tablespoons almond flour

- 1 teaspoon butter, melted

- ½ teaspoon salt

- ½ teaspoon ground turmeric

- ¼ teaspoon dried sage

Directions:

1. Mix up together grated zucchini and egg.

2. When the mixture is homogenous, add shredded Mozzarella and almond flour.

3. After this, add salt, ground turmeric, and dried sage. Mix up the mixture.

4. Preheat the instant pot on sauté mode for 2 minutes.

5. Then toss butter inside and melt it.

6. With the help of the spoon make the fritters and place them in the hot butter.

7. Saute the fritters for 3 minutes from each side.

Nutrition value/serving: calories 69, fat 4.4, fiber 1.5, carbs 4.4, protein 4

Coconut Creamy Porridge

Prep time: 5 minutes

Cooking time: 10 minutes

Servings: 6

Ingredients:

- 1 cup chia seeds

- 1 cup sesame seeds

- 2 cups of coconut milk

- 1 teaspoon salt

- 3 tablespoons Erythritol

- ½ teaspoon vanilla extract

- 3 tablespoons butter

- 1 teaspoon clove

- ½ teaspoon turmeric

Directions:

1. Combine the coconut milk, salt, Erythritol, vanilla extract, clove, and turmeric together in the pressure cooker. Blend the mixture.

2. Close the lid, and set the pressure cooker mode to "Pressure."

3. Cook the liquid for 10 minutes. Open the lid and add chia seeds and sesame seeds.

4. Stir the mixture well and close the lid. Cook for 2 minutes.

5. Remove the dish from the pressure cooker and let it chill briefly before serving.

Nutrition: calories 467, fat 42.6, fiber 11.2, carbs 18.4, protein 9.3

Chicken Dill Quiche

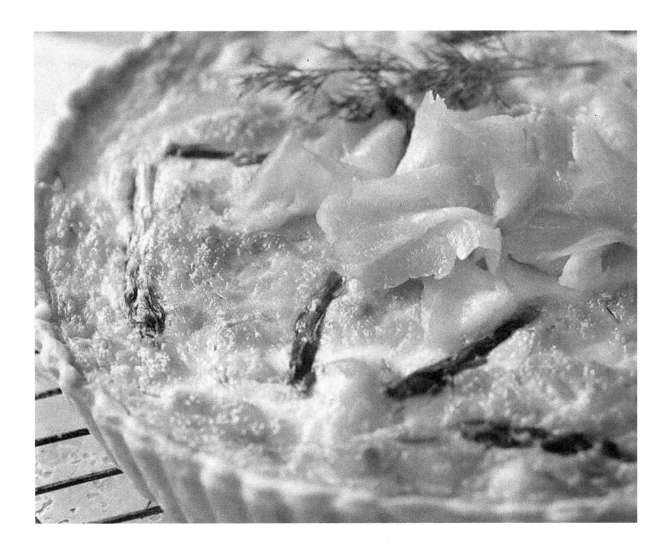

Prep time: 10 minutes

Cooking time: 30 minutes

Servings: 6

Ingredients:

- 1 pound chicken

- 1 cup dill

- 2 eggs

- 8 ounces dough

- 1 teaspoon salt

- ½ teaspoon nutmeg

- 9 ounces cheddar cheese

- ½ cup cream

- 1 teaspoon oregano

- 1 teaspoon olive oil

Directions:

1. Chop the chicken and season it with the salt, oregano, and nutmeg. Blend the mixture. Chop the dill and combine it with the chopped chicken.

2. Grate cheddar cheese. Take the round pie pan and spray it with the olive oil inside.

3. Transfer the yeast dough into the pan and flatten it well. Add the chicken mixture.

4. Whisk the eggs and add them to the quiche.

5. Sprinkle it with the grated cheese and add cream. Transfer the quiche to the pressure cooker and close the lid.

6. Set the pressure cooker mode to "Sauté," and cook for 30 minutes.

7. When the cooking time ends, remove the dish from the pressure cooker and chill it well. Cut the quiche into slices and serve it.

Nutrition: calories 320, fat 14.1, fiber 3, carbs 13.65, protein 34

Cardamom Chia Pudding

Prep time: 10 minutes

Cooking time: 15 minutes

Servings: 4

Ingredients:

- 1 cup chia seeds

- 4 tablespoons Erythritol

- 2 cups of coconut milk

- 2 tablespoons heavy cream

- 1 teaspoon butter

- 1 teaspoon cinnamon

- 1 teaspoon ground cardamom

Directions:

1. Combine the chia seeds, Erythritol, and coconut milk together in the pressure cooker.

2. Stir the mixture gently and close the lid. Set the pressure cooker mode to "Saute" and cook for 10 minutes.

3. When the cooking time ends, let the chia seeds rest little.

4. Open the pressure cooker lid and add cream, cinnamon, cardamom, and butter. Blend the mixture well using a wooden spoon.

5. Transfer the pudding to the serving bowls. Add cherry jam, if desired, and serve.

Nutrition: calories 486, fat 43.3, fiber 15.3, carbs 22.6, protein 8.8

Creamy Soufflé

Prep time: 10 minutes

Cooking time: 20 minutes

Servings: 6

Ingredients:

- 3 eggs

- 1 cup cream

- 6 ounces of cottage cheese

- 4 tablespoons butter

- ⅓ cup dried apricots

- 1 tablespoon sour cream

- 2 tablespoons sugar

- 1 teaspoon vanilla extract

Directions:

8. Whisk the eggs and combine them with cream.

9. Transfer the cottage cheese to a mixing bowl, and mix it well using a hand mixer.

10. Add the whisked eggs, butter, sour cream, sugar, and vanilla extract.

11. Blend the mixture well until smooth.

12. Add the apricots, and stir the mixture well.

13. Transfer the soufflé in the pressure cooker and close the lid. Set the pressure cooker mode to «Sauté», and cook for 20 minutes.

14. When the cooking time ends, let the soufflé cool little and serve.

Nutrition: calories 266, fat 21.1, fiber 1, carbs 11.72, protein 8

Zucchini Casserole

Prep time: 10 minutes

Cooking time: 30 minutes

Servings: 8

Ingredients:

- 6 ounces cheddar cheese

- 1 zucchini

- ½ cup ground chicken

- 4 ounces Parmesan cheese

- 3 tablespoons butter

- 1 teaspoon paprika

- 1 teaspoon salt

- 1 teaspoon basil

- 1 teaspoon cilantro

- ½ cup fresh dill

- ⅓ cup tomato juice

- ½ cup cream

- 2 red sweet bell peppers

Directions:

8. Grate cheddar cheese.

9. Chop the zucchini and combine it with the ground chicken.

10. Sprinkle the mixture with the paprika, salt, basil, cilantro, tomato juice, and cream. Stir the mixture well. Transfer it to the pressure cooker.

11. Chop the dill, sprinkle the mixture in the pressure cooker, and add the butter. Chop the Parmesan cheese and add it to the pressure cooker.

12. Chop the bell peppers and add them too. Sprinkle the mixture with the grated cheddar cheese and close the lid.

13. Set the pressure cooker mode to "Sauté", and cook for 30 minutes.

14. When the cooking time ends, let the casserole chill briefly and serve.

Nutrition: calories 199, fat 14.7, fiber 1, carbs 6.55, protein 11

Spinach Casserole

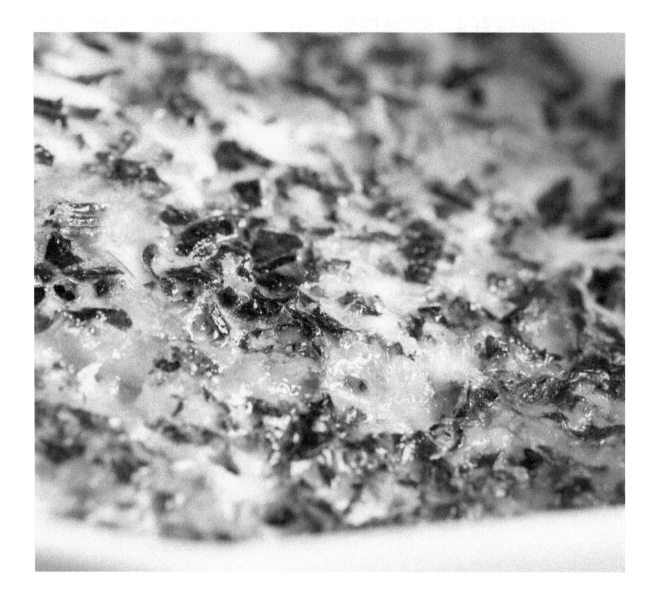

Prep time: 6 minutes

Cooking time: 6 minutes

Servings: 5

Ingredients:

- 2 cups spinach

- 8 eggs

- ½ cup almond milk

- 1 teaspoon salt

- 1 tablespoon olive oil

- 1 teaspoon ground black pepper

- 4 ounces Parmesan cheese

Directions:

7. Add the eggs to a mixing bowl and whisk them.

8. Chop the spinach and add it to the egg mixture.

9. Add the almond milk, salt, olive oil, and ground black pepper. Stir the mixture well. Transfer the egg mixture to the pressure cooker and close the lid.

10. Set the pressure cooker mode to "Steam," and cook for 6 minutes.

11. Grate the cheese. When the cooking time ends, remove the omelet from the pressure cooker and transfer it to a serving plate.

12. Sprinkle the dish with the grated cheese and serve.

Nutrition: calories 257, fat 20.4, fiber 0.9, carbs 3.4, protein 17.1

Spicy Romano Bites

Prep time: 6 minutes

Cooking time: 20 minutes

Servings: 8

Ingredients:

10 ounces Romano cheese

- 6 ounces sliced bacon

- 1 teaspoon oregano

- 5 ounces puff pastry

- 1 teaspoon butter

- 2 egg yolks

- 1 teaspoon sesame seeds

Directions:

9. Chop Romano cheese into small cubes.

10. Roll the puff pastry using a rolling pin. Whisk the egg yolks.

11. Sprinkle them with the oregano and sesame seeds.

12. Cut the puff pastry into the squares, and place an equal amount of butter on every square. Wrap the cheese cubes in the sliced bacon.

13. Place the wrapped cheese cubes onto the puff pastry squares. Make the "bites" of the dough and brush them with the egg yolk mixture.

14. Transfer the bites in the pressure cooker.

15. Close the lid, and set the pressure cooker mode to "Steam." Cook for 20 minutes.

16. When the cooking time ends, remove the dish from the pressure cooker and place on a serving dish.

Nutrition: calories 321, fat 24.4, fiber 1, carbs 10.9, protein 16

Conclusion

Being an excellent option both for immediate pot newbies and experienced instant pot users this instantaneous pot cookbook boosts your everyday cooking. It makes you appear like a professional as well as cook like a pro. Thanks to the Instantaneous Pot component, this cookbook aids you with preparing straightforward and also delicious meals for any kind of budget plan. Satisfy every person with hearty suppers, nutritive breakfasts, sweetest treats, as well as enjoyable treats. Regardless of if you cook for one or prepare bigger sections-- there's a service for any kind of feasible cooking circumstance. Enhance your methods on exactly how to cook in the most reliable means utilizing only your immediate pot, this recipe book, and some perseverance to find out quick. Valuable ideas and techniques are subtly integrated right into every dish to make your family members request new dishes over and over again. Vegetarian choices, options for meat-eaters and also very pleasing concepts to join the entire family members at the very same table. Consuming in your home is a common experience, as well as it can be so good to satisfy all together at the end of the day. Master your Immediate Pot and make the most of this brand-new experience beginning today!

CPSIA information can be obtained
at www.ICGtesting.com
Printed in the USA
LVHW020807160621
690358LV00012B/1898